GET OUTDOORS

Go Climbing!

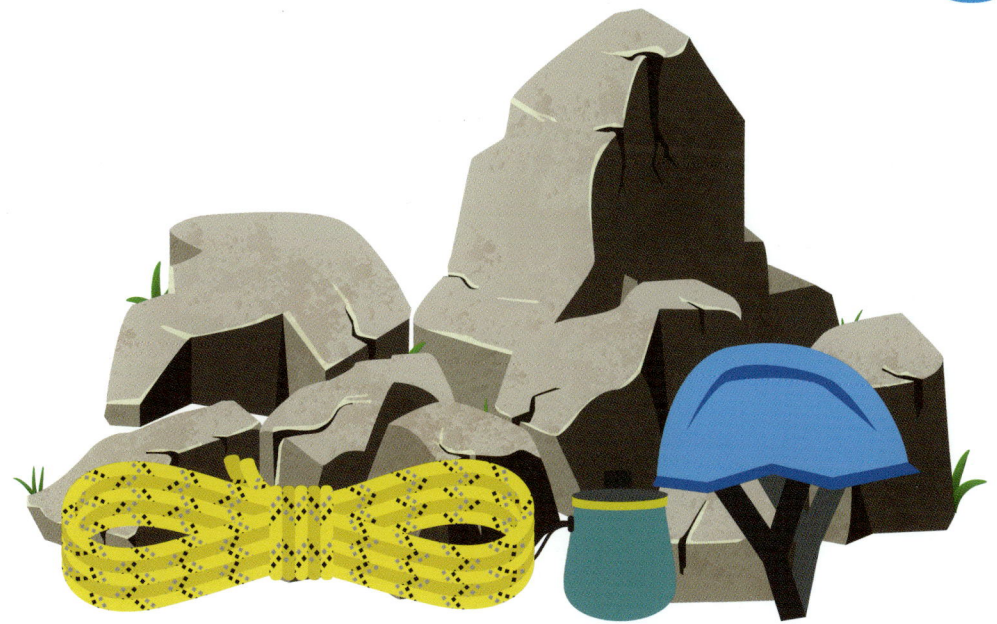

by Meghan Gottschall

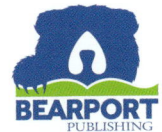

BEARPORT
PUBLISHING

Minneapolis, Minnesota

President: Jen Jenson
Director of Product Development: Spencer Brinker
Senior Editor: Allison Juda
Designer: Colin O'Dea

Library of Congress Cataloging-in-Publication Data

Names: Gottschall, Meghan, author.
Title: Go climbing! / by Meghan Gottschall.
Description: Fusion books. | Minneapolis, Minnesota : Bearport Publishing Company, 2022. | Series: Get outdoors | Includes bibliographical references and index.
Identifiers: LCCN 2021001062 (print) | LCCN 2021001063 (ebook) | ISBN 9781647479688 (library binding) | ISBN 9781647479756 (paperback) | ISBN 9781647479824 (ebook)
Subjects: LCSH: Rock climbing--Juvenile literature.
Classification: LCC GV200.2 .G67 2022 (print) | LCC GV200.2 (ebook) | DDC 796.522/3--dc23
LC record available at https://lccn.loc.gov/2021001062
LC ebook record available at https://lccn.loc.gov/2021001063

Copyright © 2022 Bearport Publishing Company. All rights reserved. No part of this publication may be reproduced in whole or in part, stored in any retrieval system, or transmitted in any form or by any means, electronic, mechanical, photocopying, recording, or otherwise, without written permission from the publisher.

For more information, write to Bearport Publishing, 5357 Penn Avenue South, Minneapolis, MN 55419. Printed in the United States of America.

Image Credits

Cover, © swinner/Shutterstock, © swinner/Shutterstock, © NEILRAS/Shutterstock; 1, © Maria Ticce/Shutterstock; 5T, © Slatan/Shutterstock; 5B, © Vitalii Matokha/Shutterstock; 6L, © Alisha Bube/Getty Images; 6R, © Alohalika/Getty Images; 7, © zhukovvvlad/Shutterstock; 8, © Anchiy/Getty Images; 9, © michelecaminati/Shutterstock; 11, © Sergey Novikov/Shutterstock; 12, © adirekjob/Shutterstock; 13, © thinair28/Getty Images; 14R, © YazanMRihan/Pixabay; 14L, © JJuni/Pixabay; 15, © Daniel Schweinert/Shutterstock; 16, © OpenClipart-Vectors/Pixabay; 17, © Erik Isakson/Getty Images; 20, © fotoVoyager/Getty Images; 21, © Nataliia Liubinetska/Shutterstock; 22, © Sylvia sooyoN/Shutterstock; 23, © Chris Dingwall/Shutterstock; Background: © Clker-Free-Vector-Images/Pixabay, © Merggy/Shutterstock, © Shirstok/Shutterstock; Elements: © Janjf93/Pixabay, © Kaliene/Pixabay, © OpenClipart-Vectors/Pixabay, © NotionPic/Shutterstock, © JungleOutThere/Shutterstock, © Colorlife/Shutterstock, © aliaksei kruhlenia/Shutterstock, © Sudowoodo/Shutterstock

CONTENTS

A Climbing Adventure............4
Gearing Up......................6
Head to Toe.....................8
Where to Go....................10
All About Bouldering...........12
What's the Problem?............14
All About Rock Climbing........16
Belay On!......................18
Mountain Climbing.............. 20
At the Top..................... 22
Glossary 24
Index.......................... 24

A CLIMBING ADVENTURE

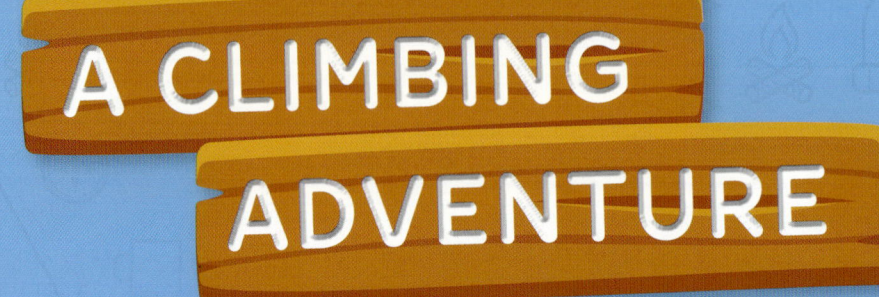

Climbing is a fun outdoor activity. You have to be strong and smart to work your way to the top. Let's go on a climbing adventure.

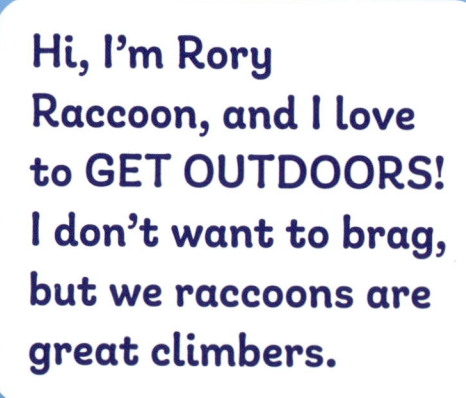

Hi, I'm Rory Raccoon, and I love to GET OUTDOORS! I don't want to brag, but we raccoons are great climbers.

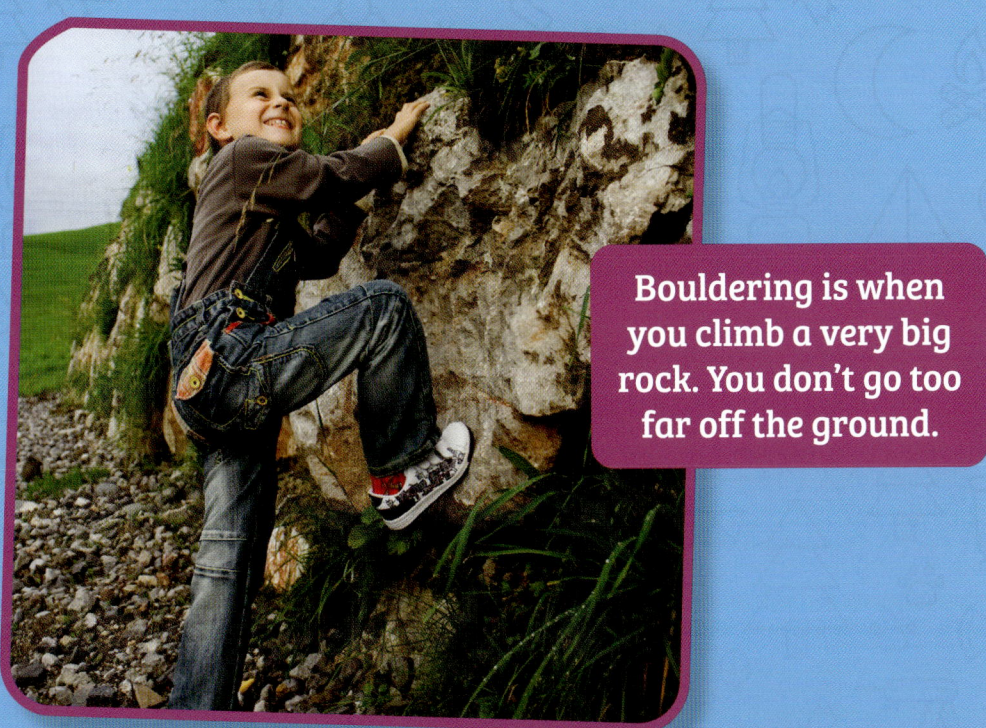

Bouldering is when you climb a very big rock. You don't go too far off the ground.

You can go even higher with rock climbing. This is because ropes keep you safe on your way up.

GEARING UP

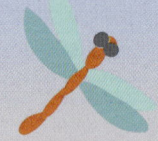

What kind of gear will you need for your climb? Bouldering doesn't need much gear. Chalk keeps your hands dry. This gives you a better **grip** on the rock. A crash pad is a thick mat that gives you a soft place to land if you fall.

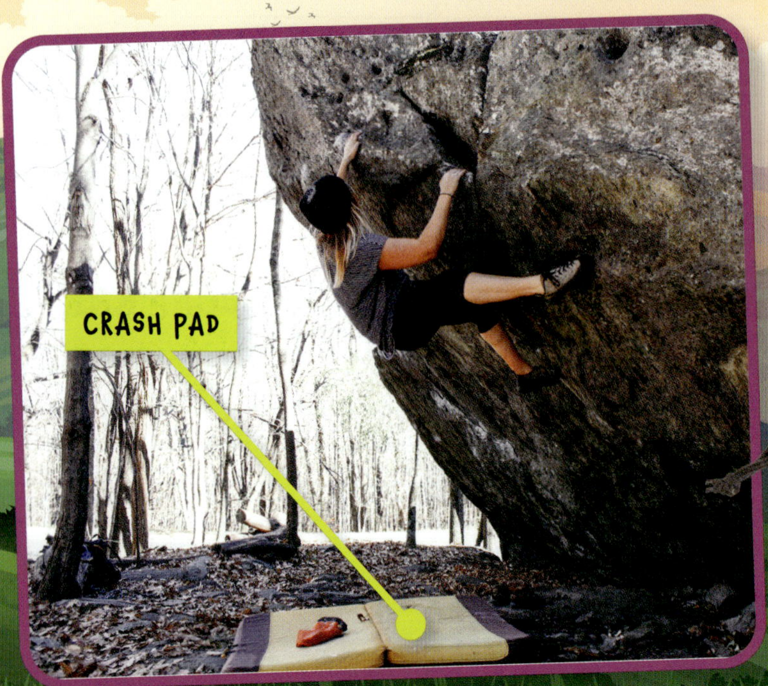

CRASH PAD

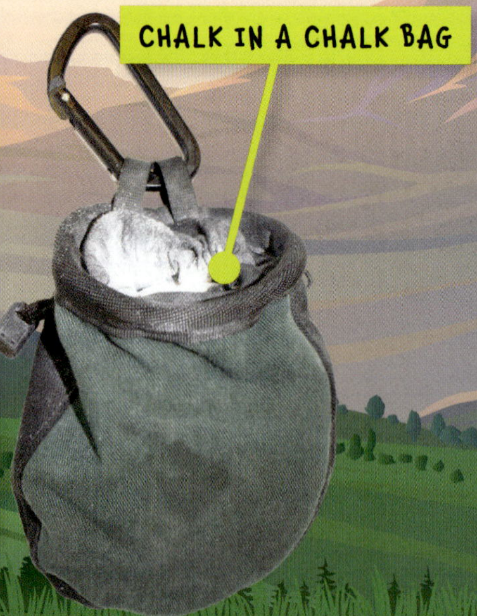

CHALK IN A CHALK BAG

For rock climbing, you need a **harness**. It goes around you, and then you attach the harness to a rope. Chalk helps for this kind of climbing, too.

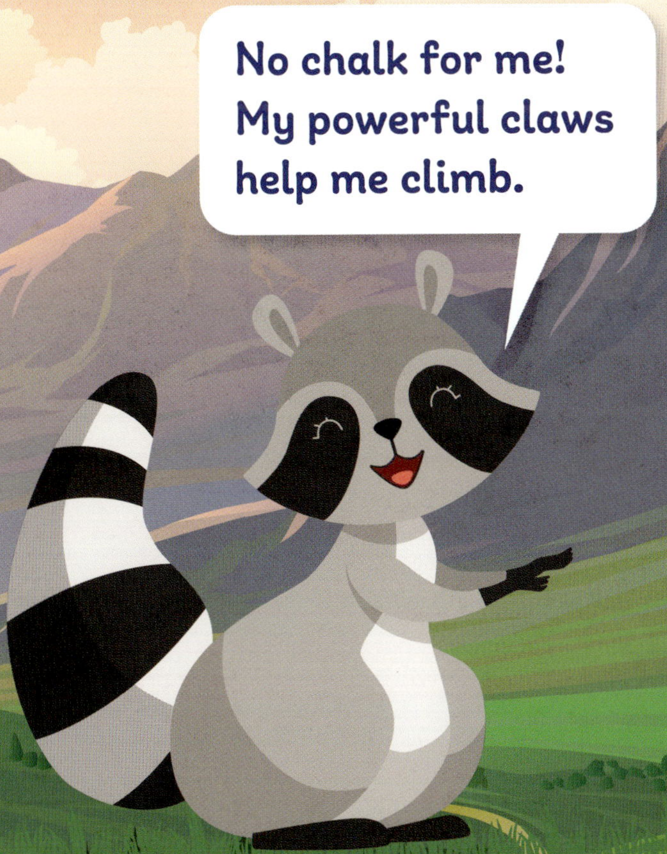

No chalk for me! My powerful claws help me climb.

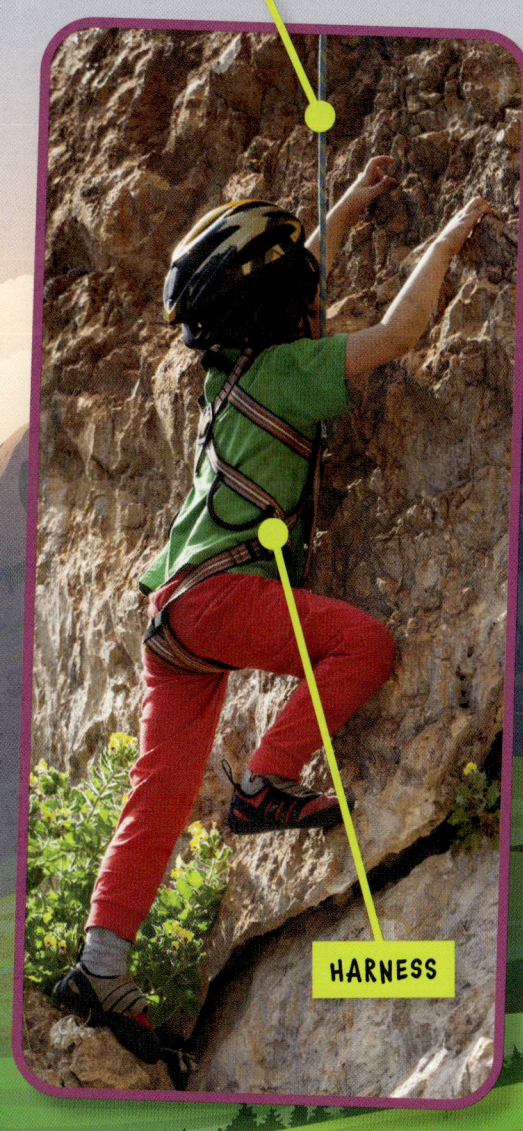

ROPE

HARNESS

HEAD TO TOE

What should you wear to go climbing? Let's start at the top. You need a climbing helmet for rock climbing. Some people wear one for bouldering, too.

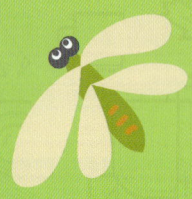

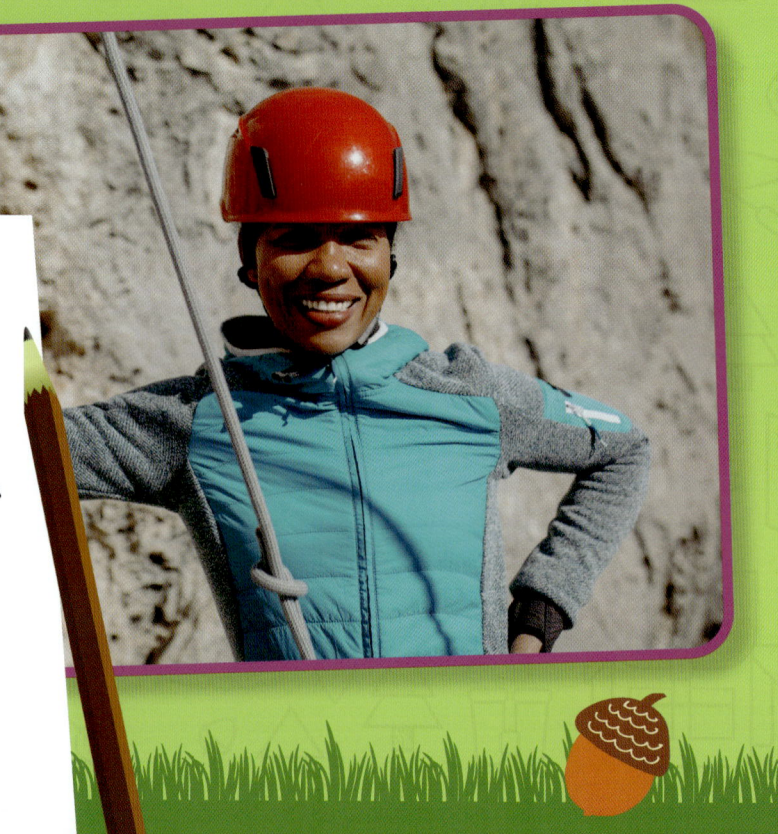

A bike helmet won't work well for climbing. A climbing helmet protects you from falling rocks in a way a bike helmet does not.

Let's make our way down to your toes. Wear climbing shoes. They should be snug but not too tight. Climbing shoes help you climb better because you can feel the rocks with your feet.

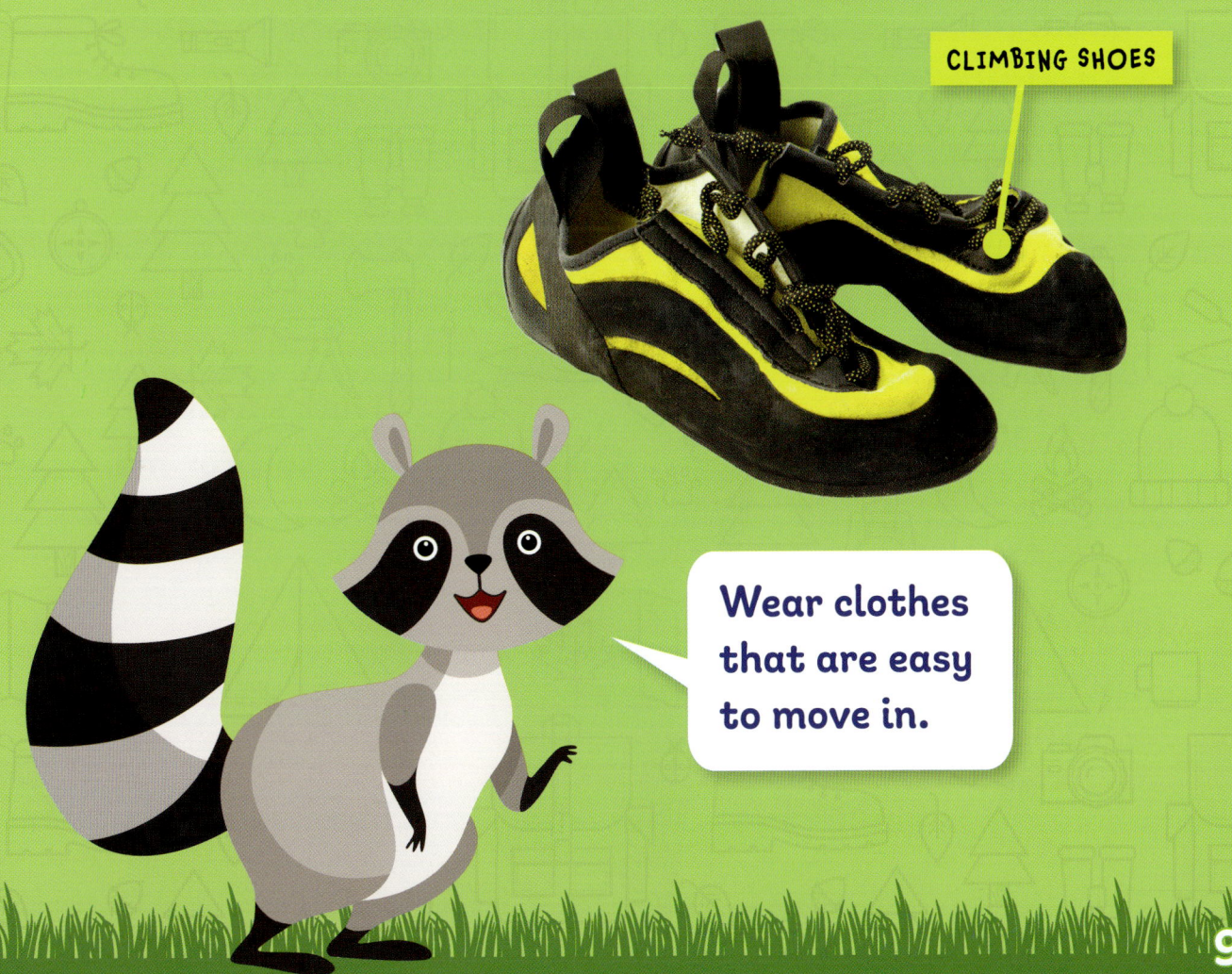

CLIMBING SHOES

Wear clothes that are easy to move in.

WHERE TO GO

Now, it's time to decide where to climb! Many local parks, **state parks**, and **national parks** have climbing areas. Look for someplace near you. Choose a climb where the ground below is flat.

The tallest outdoor climbing wall is at Basecamp Climbing Gym in Reno, Nevada. It's 164 feet (50 m) tall. That's half as tall as the Statue of Liberty!

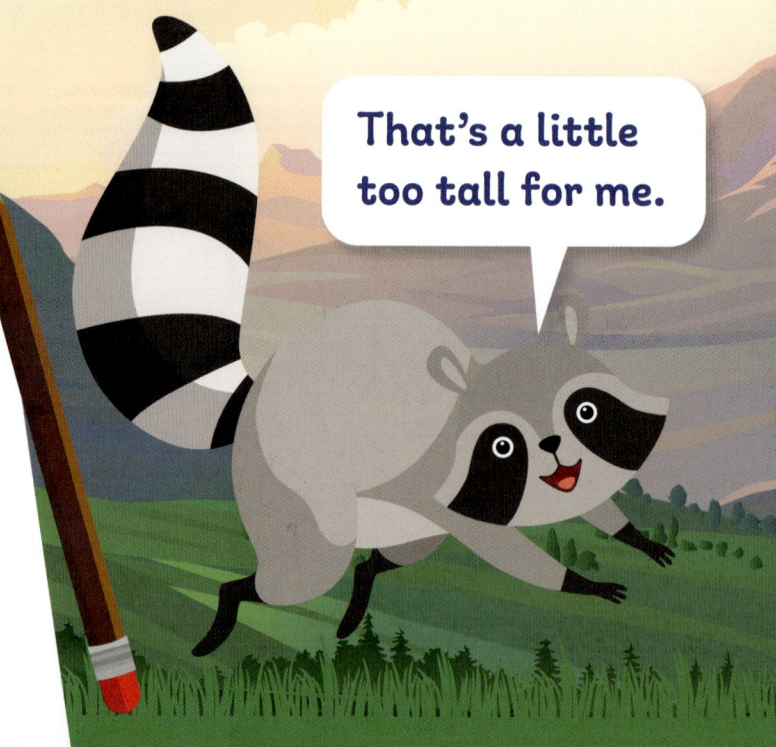

That's a little too tall for me.

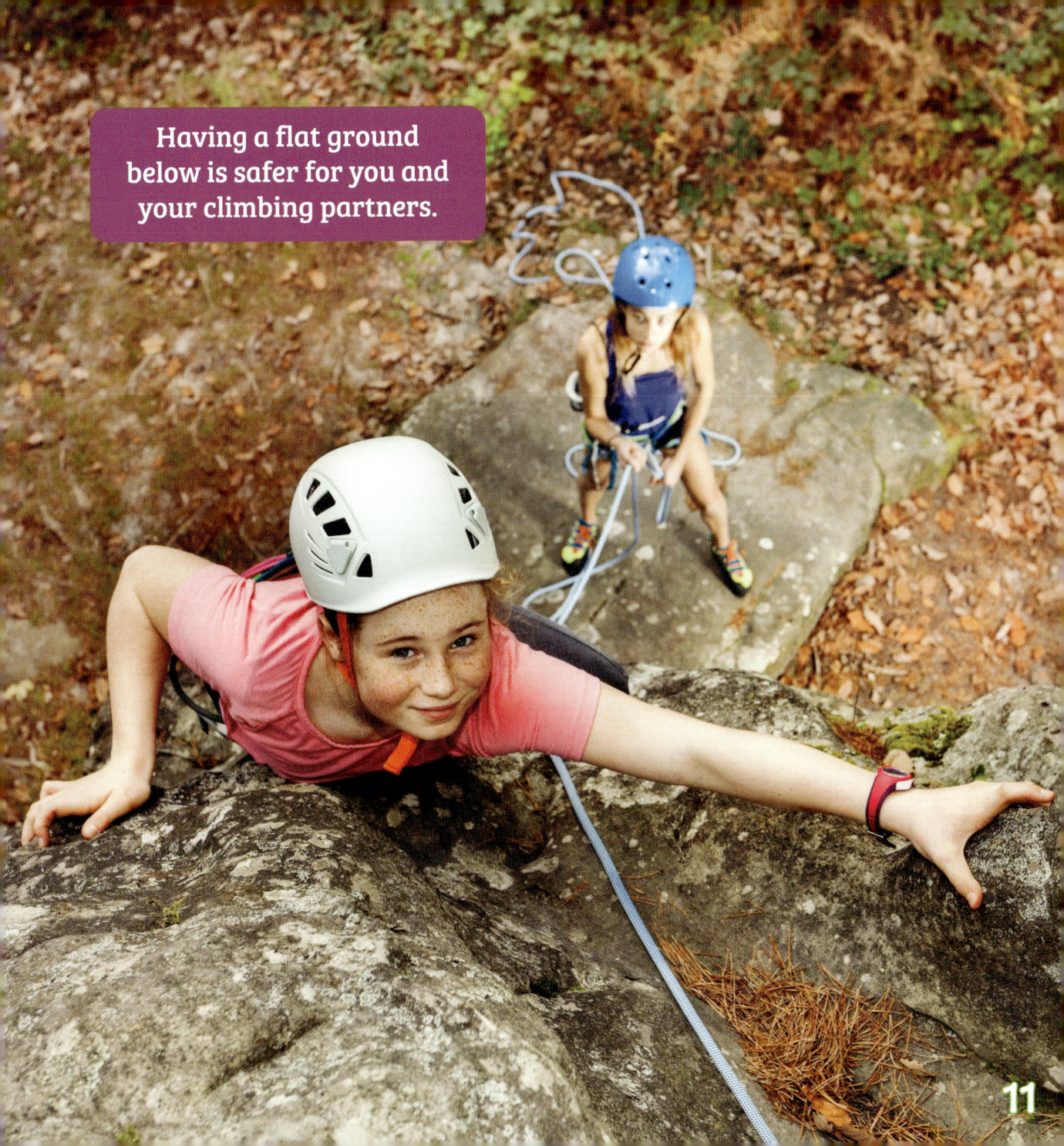
Having a flat ground below is safer for you and your climbing partners.

ALL ABOUT BOULDERING

Let's learn more about bouldering. Bouldering rocks are around 15–20 ft (4.5–6 m) high. You move up or across the rock. On human-made bouldering walls, there might be plastic places to hold and stand on.

The places where you grab with your hands are called **handholds**, and the places where you put your feet are **toeholds**.

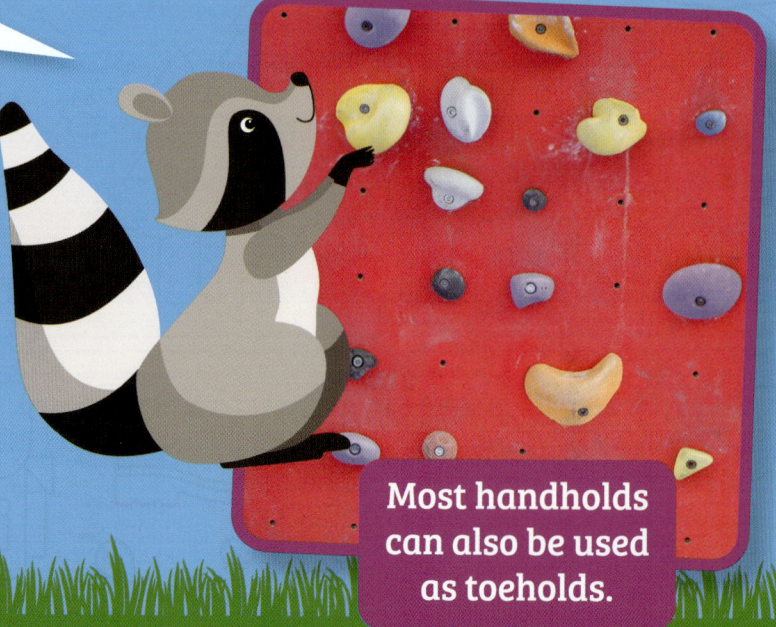

Most handholds can also be used as toeholds.

Make sure you always have an adult **spotting** you. They stand below you with their arms out. They're ready to help you if you need it.

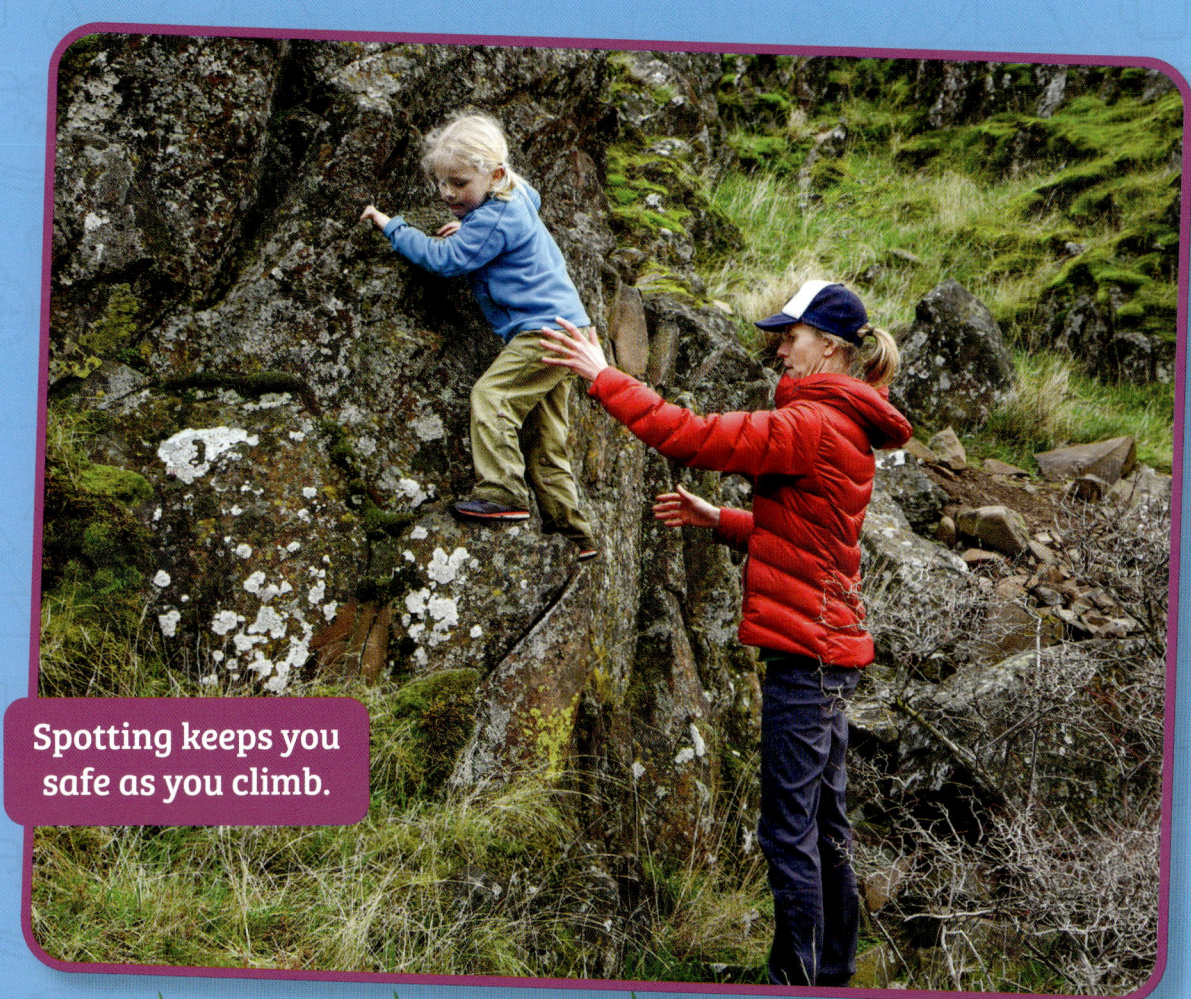

Spotting keeps you safe as you climb.

13

WHAT'S THE PROBLEM?

Bouldering is all about solving problems. Really! In bouldering, different climbing paths are called problems. Climbers must make their way from the start of the climb to the end to solve problems.

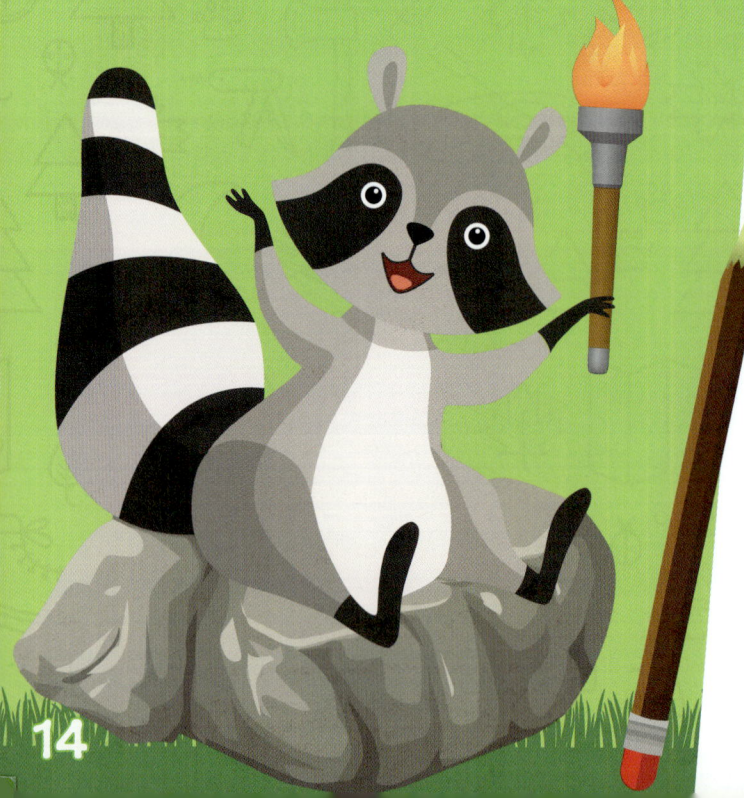

Bouldering and other sport climbing recently became Olympic sports.

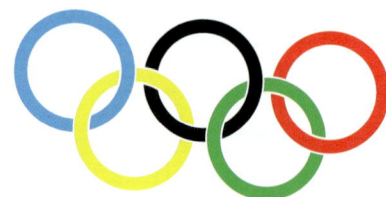

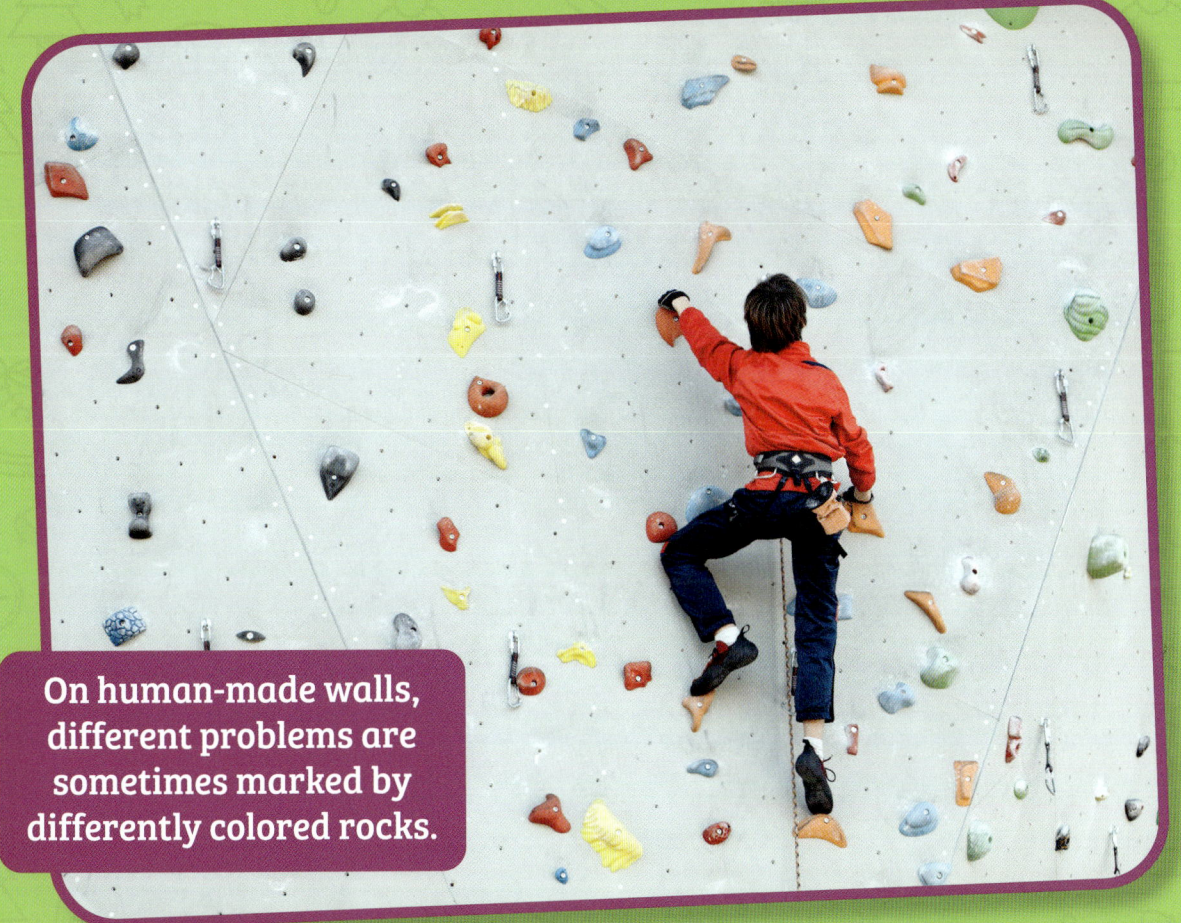

On human-made walls, different problems are sometimes marked by differently colored rocks.

Problems might be marked on the boulder or wall. Some problems are harder than others. Start with an easy one and work your way up to something harder!

ALL ABOUT ROCK CLIMBING

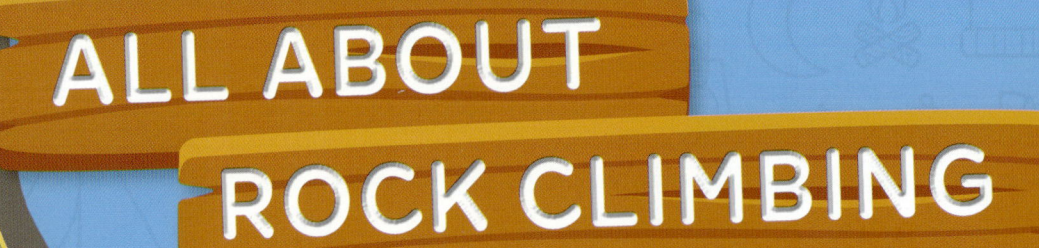

"The views up here are amazing!"

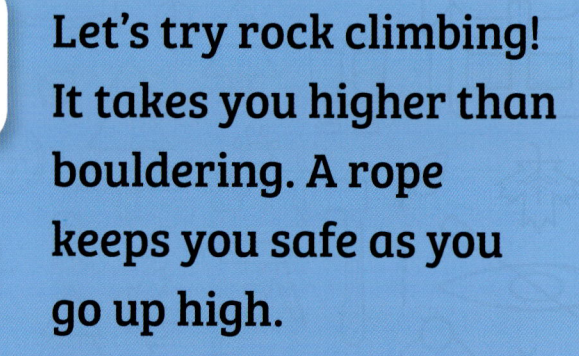

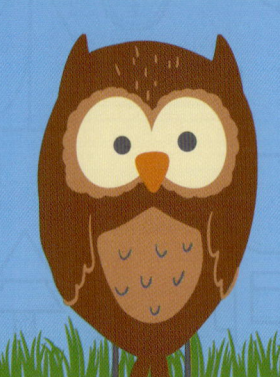

Let's try rock climbing! It takes you higher than bouldering. A rope keeps you safe as you go up high.

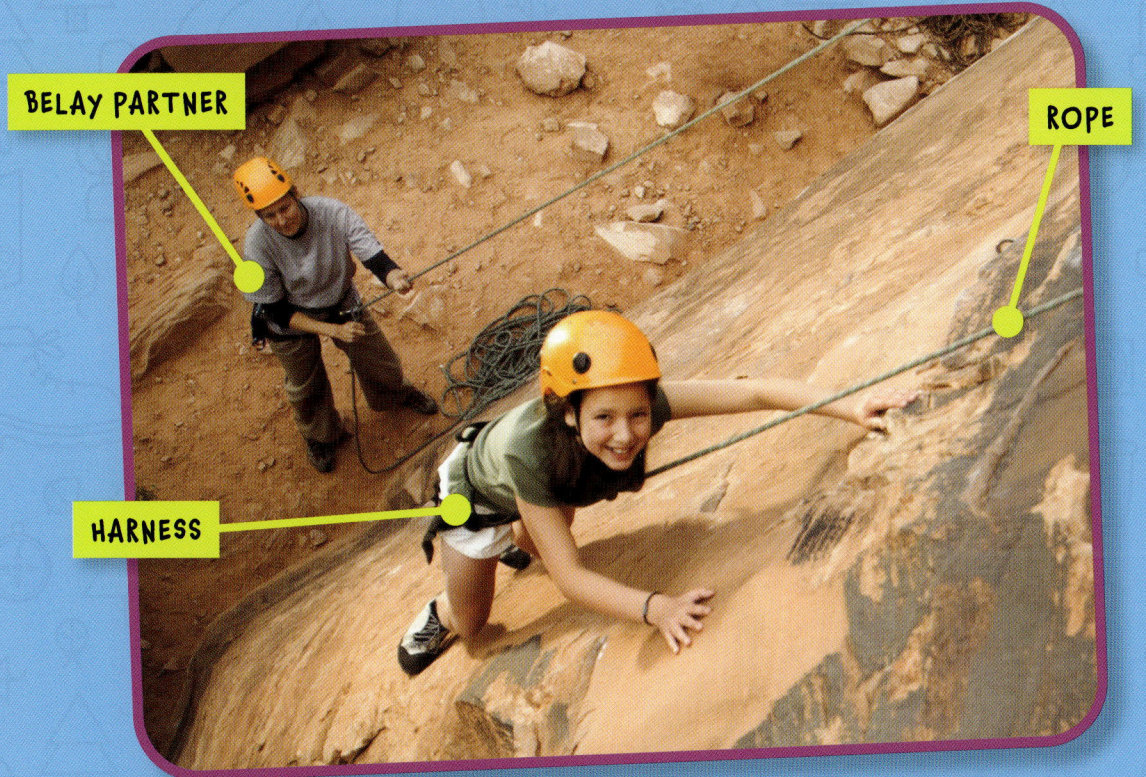

BELAY PARTNER

ROPE

HARNESS

Attach the rope to your harness. An adult should be your **belay** partner. They stay on the ground with the other end of the rope on their own harness. If you lose your grip on the wall, the rope keeps you up. Grab a handhold and start climbing!

BELAY ON!

Up rope! Slack! Belay on! Wait . . . what? It's time to learn the lingo. Telling your belay partner what you need helps you stay safe when climbing.

> Ask your partner "On belay?" to make sure they're ready for you to climb. Your partner will answer "Belay on!" Now you can start climbing.

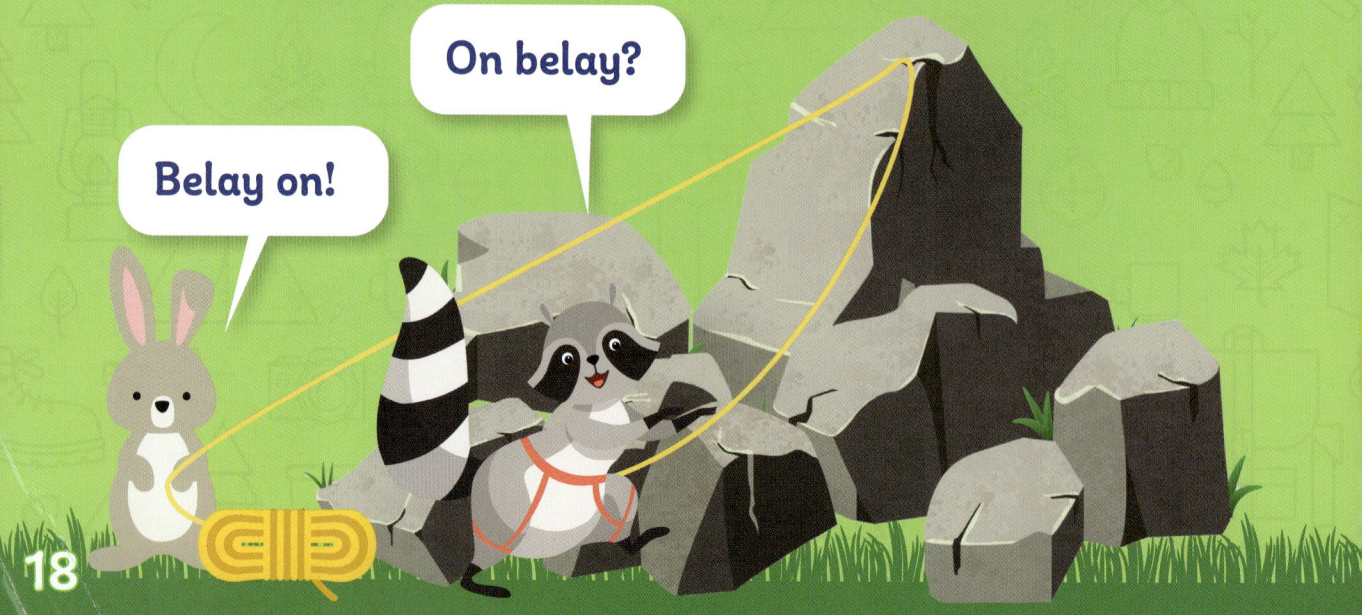

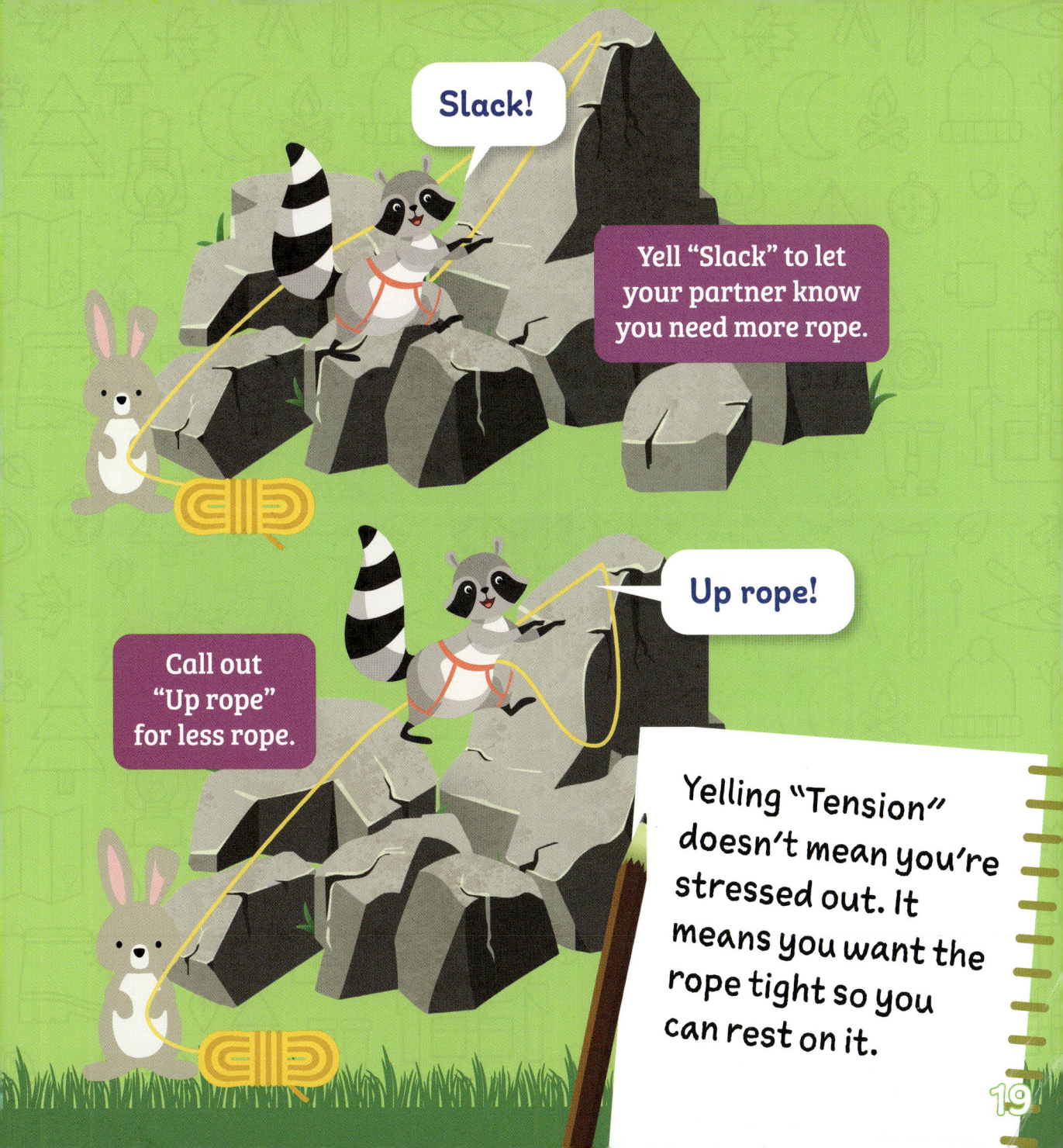

MOUNTAIN CLIMBING

Want a different view from your climb? Try mountain climbing. It often includes a mix of rock climbing and hiking.

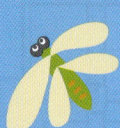

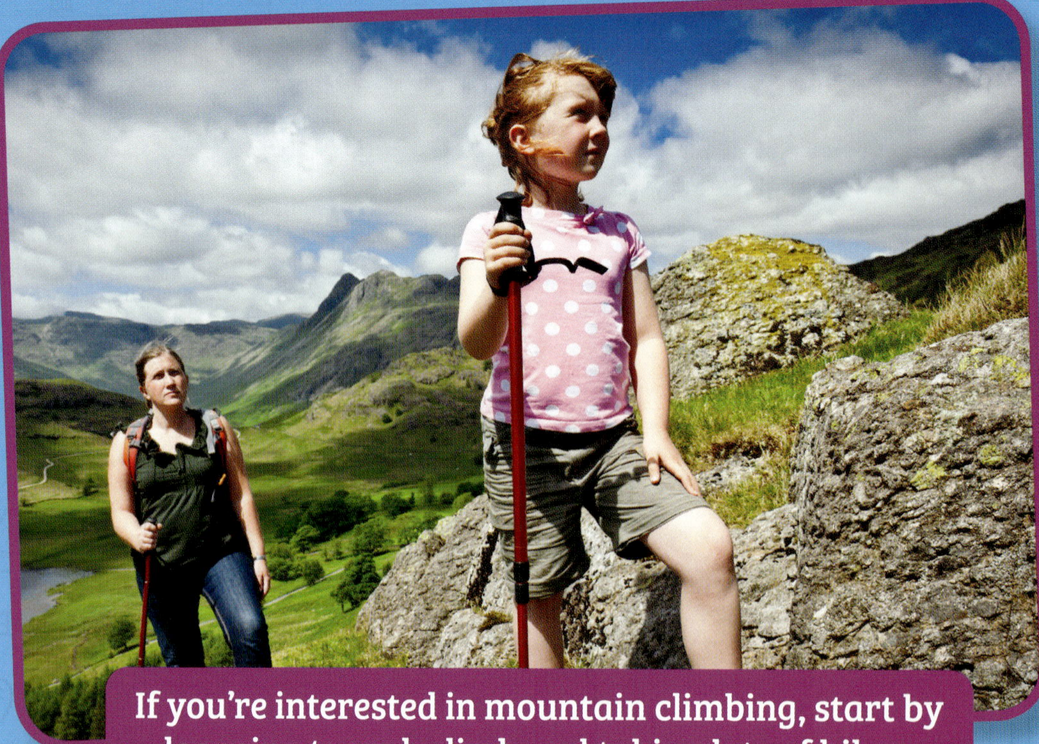

If you're interested in mountain climbing, start by learning to rock climb and taking lots of hikes.

In cold weather, mountain climbers often need special gear. It helps them climb through ice and snow.

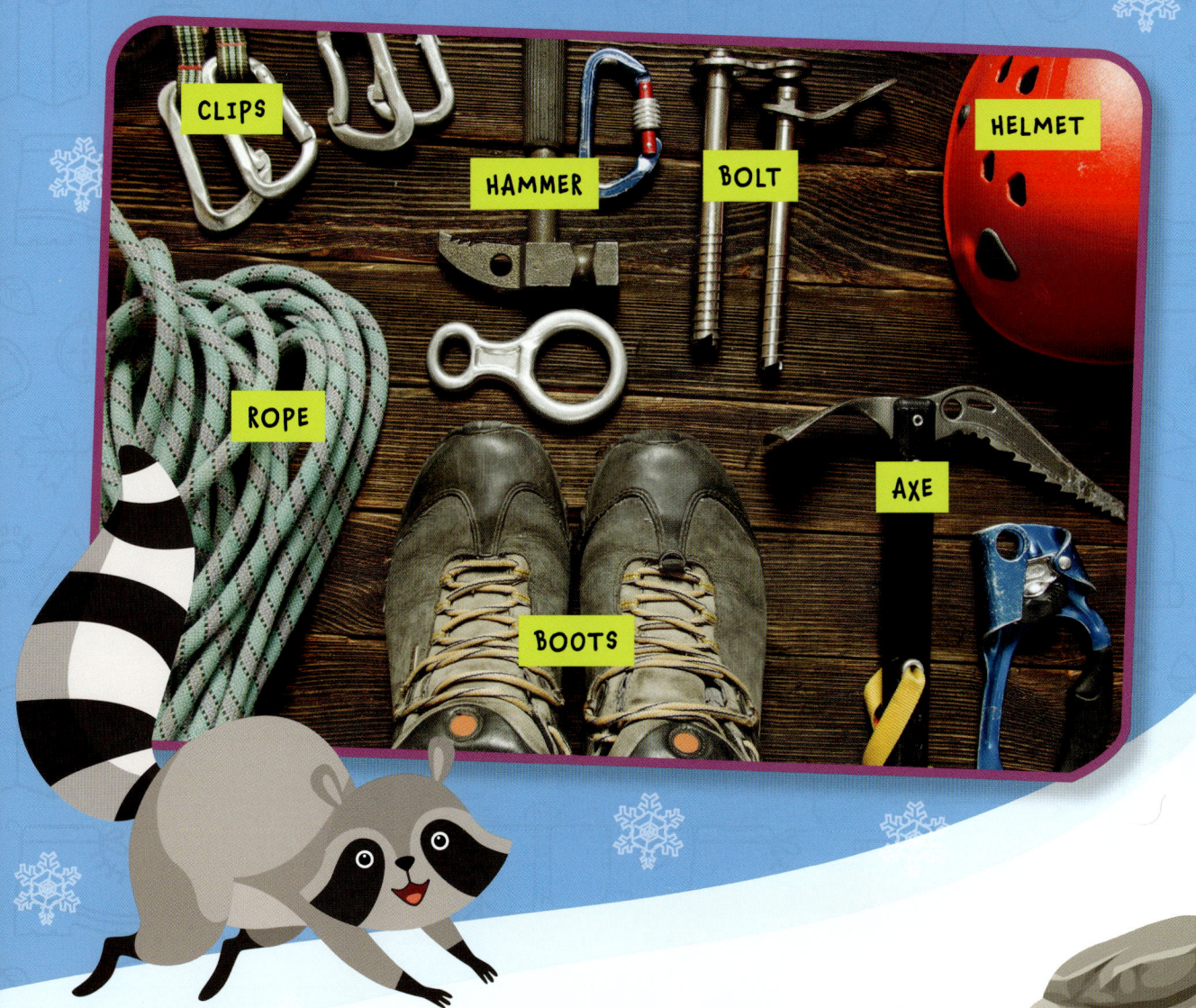

AT THE TOP

You need to be strong and smart to climb. But it's worth the hard work. Not only is it fun, but also climbing lets you spend some time outside. Where will your next climbing adventure take you?

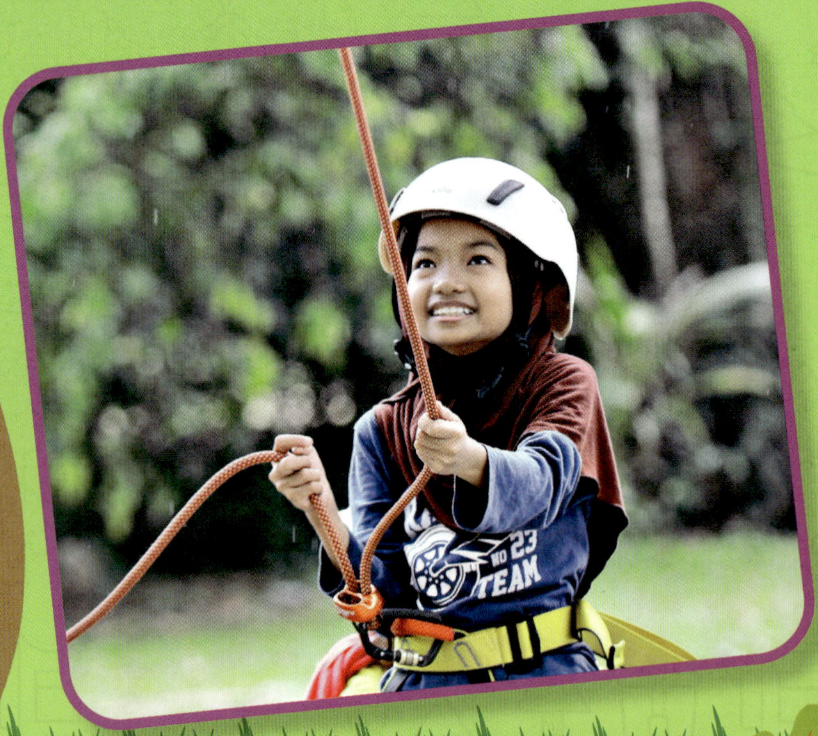

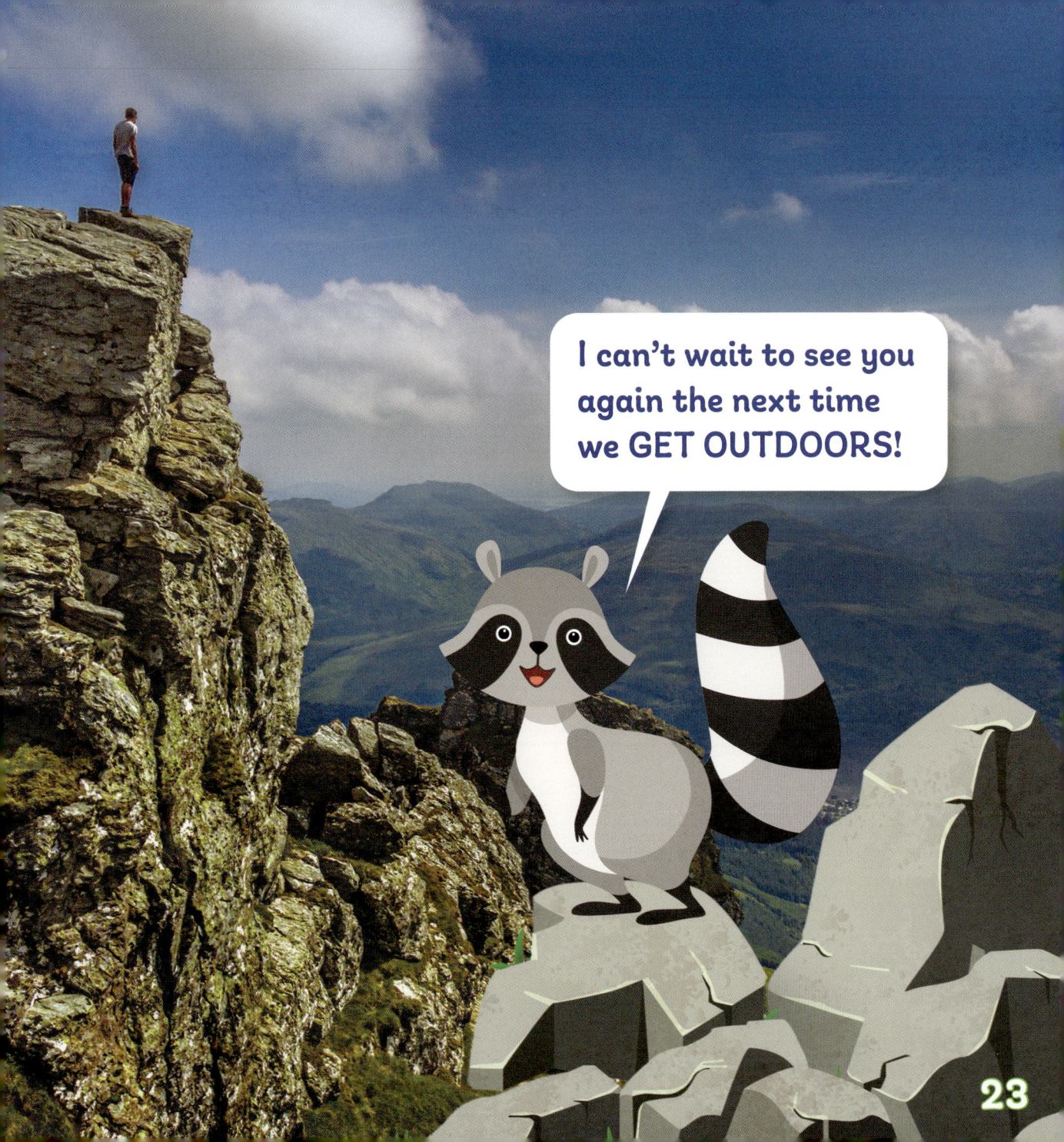

GLOSSARY

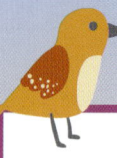

belay to attach a rope to someone to keep them safe

grip a strong hold on something

handholds parts of a rock or climbing wall that you can hold on to with your hand

harness a set of straps that attach a person to something or someone else

national parks areas of land set aside by the U.S. government to protect the animals and plants that live there

spotting watching someone doing a sport or exercising to make sure they don't get hurt

state parks areas of land set aside by state governments to protect the animals and plants that live there

toeholds parts of a rock or climbing wall where your toes can be placed

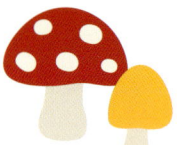

INDEX

belay 17–18
bouldering 5–6, 8, 12, 14, 16
chalk 6–7
crash pad 6

harness 7, 17
helmet 8, 21
hiking 20

mountain climbing 20–21
rock climbing 5, 7–8, 16, 20
rope 5, 7, 16–19, 21
shoes 9